Managing Complex Cases

A study guide for case managers

June Stark, RN, BSN, MEd
Della W. Webb, LCSW, CCM

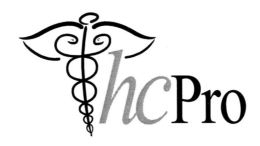

Managing Complex Cases: A study guide for case managers is published by HCPro, Inc.

Copyright 2004 HCPro, Inc.

June Stark, RN, BSN, MEd, Author
Della W. Webb, LCSW, CCM, Author
Emily Sheahan, Executive Editor
Jackie Diehl Singer, Graphic Artist
Rebecca Delaney, Associate Editor
Kelly Ahlquist, Copy Editor
Jean St. Pierre, Creative Director
Shane Katz, Cover Designer
Paul Singer, Layout Artist
Kathy Levesque, Group Publisher
Suzanne Perney, Publisher

For more information, contact:

HCPro, Inc.
200 Hoods Lane
P.O. Box 1168
Marblehead, MA 01945
Telephone: 800/650-6787 or 781/639-1872
Fax: 781/639-2982
E-mail: *customerservice@hcpro.com*

Visit HCPro at its World Wide Web sites:
www.hcmarketplace.com and www.hcpro.com.

Contents —————————————————————————

About the authors

June Stark, RN, BSN, MEd

June Stark, RN, BSN, MEd, is the director of case management at Salem Hospital and North Shore Medical Center in Salem, MA, which includes Salem and Union Hospitals. She also acts as an associate consultant for The Center of Case Management in Natick, MA. Stark was involved in the development of case management at New England Medical Center in the 1980s and worked as the director of care management at Saint Elizabeth's Medical Center in Brighton, MA.

Della W. Webb, LCSW, CCM

Della W. Webb, LCSW, CCM, is the manager of patient care coordination at Piedmont Hospital in Atlanta. Webb is a case manager with more than 25 years of experience in medical social work program administration and case management program development. Before joining Piedmont Hospital, Webb was the director of social work and discharge planning at Prince Williams Hospital Corp., in Manassas, VA.

Webb received her master's in social work from Bryn Mawr School of Social Work and Research in Pennsylvania, and her bachelor's at Morgan State University in Baltimore.

Introduction ————————————————

As a case manager you are expected to perform an intricate and challenging balancing act. While managing complex patients such as illegal immigrants, indigent patients, those with mental health or substance abuse issues, and those facing end-of-life, you are responsible for developing a safe discharge plan while also working to reduce length of stay (LOS) and resource utilization—certainly not an easy task.

Managing Complex Cases: A study guide for case managers is a multifaceted tool designed to help case managers tackle these complicated discharge challenges. In this guide you will find 12 complex cases carefully chosen by practicing case managers that represent various types of patients that they see in their facilities. These cases are real-life scenarios, with only the identifying factors changed, giving case managers an authentic snapshot of how colleagues handled complex cases.

This guide can be used by all levels of case managers and is meant to spark conversations between case management colleagues, case managers and their directors, and new case managers and their preceptors. Following each case, you'll find areas for jotting down resources and ideas that come up during a discussion with your peers—making this guide a reference tool that you can revisit when faced with similar complex cases.

Another tried and tested case management tool provided in this book is the HAL model, a case management competency assessment tool developed by Della Webb, LCSW, CCM, manager of patient care coordination at Piedmont Hospital in Atlanta. Webb created the model for case managers to use to assess their strengths, weaknesses, and any cultural or life experiences they bring to a complex case. Using this competency assessment tool increases your awareness before you begin a case, which in turn increases your productivity and efficiency. Complete the HAL model after reading each of the cases in this guide to see where you excel and where you can improve.

For more information about using the guide to train case managers, read the instructor guide included in this packet. This book offers case managers two continuing education (CE) credits from the Commission for Case Manager Certification.

After completing this study guide, case managers should be able to

- describe strategies to manage complicated patient cases to balance cost and efficiency and reduce patient LOS

- assess their strengths and weaknesses using the HAL model

- identify community resources and programs that are available for patients with complicated issues

Use this study guide as a mirror to hold up to your own practice and reflect on how you would handle these complex cases. Share your ideas and resources with your colleagues as you become more adept at balancing patient safety, LOS, and cost efficiency.

How to use the HAL model ———————————

Background

Length of stay has decreased at Atlanta's Piedmont Hospital, and attitudes about complex cases are changing. "Bring it on" is the new philosophy in Piedmont's case management department thanks to an assessment tool called the HAL model created by Della W. Webb, LCSW, CCM, manager of patient care coordination at Piedmont.

This section will show you how to apply this assessment tool to the complex cases you face. Use it whenever you are confronted with a challenging case. It will only take a few minutes, but it is crucial to the discharge planning process and to improved productivity among case managers, says Webb.

This section provides a case study that illustrates how to apply the assessment tool and use it to enhance your ability to manage challenging cases. Eventually, you may change how you view complex cases.

The one-page scoring tool appears at the end of this section.

Note: Webb advises care coordination directors and managers to include the tool in annual evaluations. See the final section, "Evaluation," for details.

Thou shall honor HAL

HAL stands for the following:

H = High to very effective (score of >75%)
A = Average to moderately effective (score of 50%–75%)
L = Low to minimally effective (score of <50%)

Use this model to assess strengths and weaknesses in four fundamental components of effective case management:

1. Professional and personnel comfort with the case (your PC-1 rating)
2. Professional competency (your PC-2 rating)
3. Consultation (your C-1 rating)
4. Collaboration (your C-2 rating)

Add these four ratings to reach effective case management:

PC-1 + PC-2 + C-1 + C-2 = *Effective* CM

Your level of case management effectiveness will determine your definition of case complexity. The more complex a case seems to you at first, the less competent you may feel in handling it. But as you gain case management competency and learn how to tap into new resources through this model—such as community options, insurance options, and internal contacts—you will invariably view fewer cases as complex.

The HAL model—step by step

Professional comfort
Your score in this component represents one-quarter of your overall rating.

Step I:
Review the patient's case and history.

Step II:
Write down or consider your strengths, weaknesses, experiences, and attitudes in conjunction with the following factors. We've provided the questions to help you understand the meaning behind these factors. **Note:** The sample case study after this section can further help you. After the first few times you run through this exercise, you'll begin to remember it easily and be able to quickly assess the following factors:

- Professional/objectivity
  - *Do you think you have the ability to be neutral in handling this case?*

- Personal values and ethics
  - *What's important to you?*

- Cultural and religious influence
    - *What makes up your personal background?*

- Life experiences and maturity
    - *Have you had limited experiences with different age groups and cultures?*

- Personality type
    - *Are you a perfectionist, a type A? Will that create stress for you in managing this case?*

- Family history/dynamics
    - *Do your family background and experience influence your professional comfort with this case?*

Step III:
Now, based on your honest assessment, rate your professional comfort level according to this scale:

High = 25%, Average = 15%, Low = 5%

You might give yourself a 15% average rating if, for example, you believe you're comfortable in managing the case but have some concerns about your objectivity. This is not a perfect science; it's more important to be honest. Your manager isn't grading you on this per se; it's a tool for you.

Professional competency
Your score in this component represents one-quarter of your overall rating.

Steps I and II:
Take the same steps you took for professional comfort above, reviewing the case and assessing your strengths and weaknesses for the following—only this time, base your overall rating on your professional competency with the specific case at hand.

For example, if the case involves a Spanish-speaking patient with diabetes, schizophrenia, and medication issues who was raised in the inner-city, assess your knowledge and experience with these factors:

- Clinical knowledge and skills
    - *What do you know about diabetes, schizophrenia, and the medication used to treat both conditions?*

- Professional training and education
    - *Have you attended any inservices or seminars concerning the patient's diagnoses? What is your formal nursing and case management training?*

- Licensure and certification/code of ethics
    - *Refer to conditions of nursing licensure and the Case Management Society of America's Standards of Practice.*

- Resources for gaining knowledge
    - *Do you have mentors or colleagues you can call for ideas?*

- Skills of your manager or supervisor
    - *Managers should not avoid complex cases—if yours does, rate your professional competency as low under this factor.*

- Case experiences with these patients and populations
    - *Can you speak Spanish and have you worked with patients from the inner-city before?*

Step III:
Rate your professional competency level according to this scale:

High = 25%, Average = 15%, Low = 5%

You might give yourself a 5% average rating if, for example, you lack the training and experience for the specific case.

These next two sections should help you figure out whether you have enough resources and experts to help you manage the case and assess your willingness and attitudes about seeking help.

Consultation
Your score in this component represents one-quarter of your overall rating.

Step I:
Review the patient's case and history.

Step II:
Write down or onsider your strengths, weaknesses, and experiences for the following factors:

- Mentor or mentorship
  - *Have you been a mentor or done a preceptorship with someone on this type of case?*

- Supervision/case conferences
  - *Have you ever supervised or discussed a similar case in a case conference with fellow case managers?*

- Whom you counsel or seek counsel from
  - *Are you good at finding help, and willing to seek it? Do you have the contacts do so?*

Step III:
Rate your overall consultation level according to this scale:

High = 25%, Average = 15%, Low = 5%

You might give yourself a 25% rating if, for example, you have mentored others on a similar case.

Collaboration
Your score in this component represents one-quarter of your overall rating.

Step I:
Review the patient's case and history.

Step II:
Write down or simply consider your strengths, weaknesses, and experiences for the following factors:

- Interdisciplinary/multidisciplinary team meetings
  - *How often do you attend and contribute to multidisciplinary team meetings?*

- Ability to work together for continuity of care
  - *How well do you work with professionals from other disciplines?*

- Your ability to team up for desired goals and services
  - *Are you more of a loner when you manage cases? If so, rate your score on this last factor as low.*

Step III:
Rate your overall consultation level according to this scale:

High = 25%, Average = 15%, Low = 5%

You might give yourself a 5% rating if you prefer to work independently and feel unwilling or uncomfortable teaming up with others. That alone may be enough, in your view, to give yourself a low score. Again, think of this exercise as a way to save you time and to help your patients.

Case study using the HAL model

A case manager was given this case:

Female patient, advanced AIDS

Patient, 35, has not told her family and friends about her bisexual lifestyle. She lives alone and has two children. She's very weak with mobility and experiences some confusion. She's on medical leave from her job. She needs assistance with her activities of daily living (ADL) and mobility. Finances are a major concern. Her insurance, Blue Cross, denied three days of her hospital stay, and she is not currently meeting intensity of service criteria for discharge.

Key factors:

- Refuses alternative housing

- Refuses to let you contact family or friends

- Noncompliant with her AIDS medication because of cost

- Seems to be in denial about her diagnosis

- Diagnosed at age 25

- Shares care of her elementary school-age children with their father

- Appears too confused at times to be able to personally follow up with community resources

- Needs a walker

- Only receiving 75% of her salary because she's on medical leave

Length of stay:

- Has seven-day LOS; the last three days are denied by Blue Cross

HAL Model assessment

The following is the case manager's assessment:

1. Professional comfort (PC-1)

Professional objectivity:

- Admits to homophobia

- Displays strong emotions with patient's denial of AIDS and the risk that presents to society

- Believes many people with AIDS still have unprotected sex, which bothers the case manager

Personal values and ethics:

- Case manager is a promoter of community health and wellness programs

- She feels she has a strong work ethic

Cultural and religious influences:

- Views homosexuality as immoral

- Doesn't believe that AIDS and homosexuality is present in her community

Life experiences and maturity:

- Married 15 years, no children

- Supports AIDS awareness, education, and testing

Personality:

- Type A, describes herself as "obsessed"

Family history and dynamics:

- Says no one in her family minds his or her own business

H = 25%   A = 15%   L = 5%

2. Professional competency (PC-2)

Clinical knowledge:

- Employed two years as a case manager at the hospital

- Limited experience working with AIDS patients

- Good patient assessment skills

Education:

- Received training on the defense mechanism of denial and grief and loss issues

- Bachelor of science and registered nurse (RN)

Licensure and certification/code of ethics:

- Follows nursing code of ethics

- Working toward her certified case manager (CCM) credential

Resource knowledge base:

- Aware of local and related resources and services

- Knowledge of AIDS disease management and AIDS medications

Case experiences, patients, populations:

- Limited experience with AIDS patients

- Felt hospital didn't have enough counseling services

- Some education on disease stages and hospice

H = 25%   (A =15%)   L = 5%

3. Consultation (C-1)

Mentor or mentorship:

- Mentors/preceptor to other case managers

Supervision/case conferences:

- Discussed the case with her manager

- Presented the case during group supervision meeting (unit rounds)

- Consulted with risk management

- Never consulted insurer

- Knew that because the patient was confused there was some risk in sending her home; wanted to protect the hospital and the patient

Whom you counsel or seek counsel from:

- Has a clinical advisor

- Employee Assistance Program/private counselor

H = 25%   (A =15%)   L = 5%

4. Collaboration (C-2)

Interdisciplinary/multidisciplinary team meetings:

- Presented case at unit rounds

Work together/join forces for continuity of care:

- Collaborated with physician and unit RN

- After guidance from her manager, requested the help of an insurer-contracted case manager

Team up for desired goals and services:

- Has made referrals to home health and AIDS case management services
  (The patient felt that no one in home health would recognize her, so she felt more comfortable going this route)

- Has made referrals to adult protective services at discharge

H = 25%   (A =15%)   L = 5%

Scoring

Case manager's *initial score* with AIDS case

Pre-case

PC-1 =	5%
PC-2 =	15%
C-1 =	15%
C-2 =	15%
Total =	**50%**

The case manager's HAL score shows moderate effectiveness with the AIDS case.

After honestly assessing her strengths and weaknesses, the case manager knew in what areas to seek assistance from her director and became aware of her cultural and religious beliefs that would influence the management of this patient's care and discharge.

Case manager's HAL score after the AIDS case

PC-1 =	15% (gained comfort and awareness)
PC-2 =	25% (conducted Internet research to learn more about the patient's diseases and how they would affect her attitudes and prognosis)
C-1 =	25%
C-2 =	25%
Total =	**90%**

Highly effective with AIDS cases with continued use of HAL model

Evaluation
For directors and supervisors

The HAL model assessment is more than a tool for effective case management; it's a great method for directors to evaluate staff and measure their productivity. Use it to help you evaluate your case managers. Try the following:

- Train staff on how to use the model.

- Conduct regular team meetings to review complex cases and have case managers share their results to educate other staff.

- Ask staff to share an example of a low HAL score and how they rated themselves after the case.

- Ask case managers to keep a file of their HAL assessments and review these files periodically.

- Set goals for case managers with initial assessments with scores of <50%.

- Discuss and record on a performance review sheet what case managers can do to improve their scores and what you as a director/supervisor will do to help them achieve their goals. Hold quarterly follow-up meetings to discuss progress.

- Review the results based on the assessments and LOS data on the specific complex cases. Discuss cases and note progress and barriers to success with the case managers.

- Use this evaluation as one piece of the overall case management effectiveness review.

HAL MODEL ASSESSMENT
For complex case management

H = High to very effective (score of >75%)
A = Average to moderately effective (score of 50%–75%)
L = Low to minimally effective (score of <50%)

Professional comfort (PC-1)
H = 25% A = 15% L = 5%

Professional objectivity
Personal values and ethics
Cultural and religious influence
Life experiences and maturity
Personality type
Family history/dynamics

PC-1 score = _____

Professional competency (PC-2)
H = 25% A = 15% L = 5%

Clinical knowledge and skills
Professional training and education
Licensure and certification/code of ethics
Resource knowledge and management
Skills of your manager or supervisor
Case experiences/patients and populations

PC-2 score = _____

Consultation (C-1)
H = 25% A = 15% L = 5%

Mentor/mentorship
Supervision/case conferences
Whom you counsel/seek counsel from

C-1 score = _____

Collaboration (C-2)
H = 25% A = 15% L = 5%

Interdisciplinary/multidisciplinary meetings
Teamwork for continuity of care
Team up for desired goals

C-2 score = _____

Score: PC-1 + PC-2 + C1 + C2 = _____%

Ethics consult helps convince a difficult physician to implement a plan of care

The problem

Mrs. Brown is a 68-year-old patient who is comatose, post-ventricular fibrillation cardiac arrest, and on day five of her stay in the medical intensive care unit of a large, metropolitan teaching hospital. The case manager approaches the patient's physician, Dr. D., daily since Mrs. Brown's admission. She requests a plan, but the physician will not provide one—despite the fact that the patient shows no significant signs of improvement.

Instead, Dr. D. speaks only of continuing medical intervention. "I am going to do everything possible for Mrs. Brown," he says to the patient's husband and daughter. "I see no end to this case."

The case manager notices that the family seems to hang onto every word of hope expressed by the physician, and she believes that this presentation is not in the best interest of the family because the patient's prognosis remains unclear.

The case manager's approach

Frustrated by the multiple concerns presented by this case—including the absence of a plan of care, the lack of an established realistic prognosis, the ongoing encouragement to the family in a case that may prove to be futile, and the high utilization of clinical resources—the case manager turns to her peers.

When her peers cannot offer any suggestions, she has no choice but to move the case up the chain of command to her case management director and her physician medical advisor.

Together, they review the case and decide that the medical advisor should intervene on a physician-to-physician level. This type of exchange often proves successful, but, in this case, Dr. D. is adamant about continuing care despite the prognosis.

In the course of the discussion with the medical advisor, Dr. D. also mentions that his own mother is the same age as the patient. It becomes clear that a definite conflict in values exists between Dr. D. and the case management team. The next step is to seek a consult with the hospital's ethics committee.

The case manager wastes no time requesting an ethics consult. If a request is inappropriate or too early, it usually prolongs a case. However, with this patient, she believes she has taken all the necessary steps prior to requesting the consult, and, in the long run, it will benefit everyone involved.

The outcome

When the ethics committee convenes, representatives from the patient's caregiving and spiritual teams attend all the sessions. Dr. D. remains reluctant to terminate the care throughout most of the ethics review process, but gradually becomes more open to the inevitable outcome of this case.

At the conclusion of the review, Dr. D. is able to develop a reasonable plan of care that considers the complexity of the clinical case, the family's needs, and the patient's wishes. The case manager is now able to coordinate care and quality while working toward achieving the expected outcome of this case.

Resources

Name and contact information of medical advisor:

_____

_____

Hospital ethics committee contact information:

_____

_____

Process your facility uses to request an ethics consult:

_____

_____

Other resources:

_____

_____

HAL MODEL ASSESSMENT
For complex case management

H = High to very effective (score of >75%)
A = Average to moderately effective (score of 50%–75%)
L = Low to minimally effective (score of <50%)

Professional comfort (PC-1)
H = 25% A = 15% L = 5%

Professional objectivity
Personal values and ethics
Cultural and religious influence
Life experiences and maturity
Personality type
Family history/dynamics

PC-1 score = _____

Professional competency (PC-2)
H = 25% A = 15% L = 5%

Clinical knowledge and skills
Professional training and education
Licensure and certification/code of ethics
Resource knowledge and management
Skills of your manager or supervisor
Case experiences/patients and populations

PC-2 score = _____

Consultation (C-1)
H = 25% A = 15% L = 5%

Mentor/mentorship
Supervision/case conferences
Whom you counsel/seek counsel from

C-1 score = _____

Collaboration (C-2)
H = 25% A = 15% L = 5%

Interdisciplinary/multidisciplinary meetings
Teamwork for continuity of care
Team up for desired goals

C-2 score = _____

Score: PC-1 + PC-2 + C1 + C2 = _____%

Considering the patient's best interest, payment, and bed capacity while managing a case

The problem

A husband and wife, ages 92 and 89 respectively, come to the emergency department (ED) one evening. The husband is in good health, and the wife has mild dementia with periods of clearing. Both patients ambulate well without assistance.

The elderly couple live with one of their daughters who acts as the primary caregiver. The visiting nurses association and the state elder services program provide further support to the couple.

The couple's son brought them to the ED. The son has requested custodial placement from Elder Protective Services, saying his sister abused his parents. He is also seeking a court order to remove their parents from his sister's home. The son has contacted a lawyer who is directing his actions.

By bringing his parents to the ED, the son hopes a physician, who is unfamiliar with his parents, will admit them for a three-night stay so Medicare will cover placement in a nursing home.

A psychiatrist assesses the couple in the ED and states that there are no active psychiatric issues at that time.

The case manager's approach

The case manager is called to the ED to determine whether the couple needs hospital-level care, and whether a three-night stay is justified. She is aware that the ED is almost full and that the in-house hospital beds are limited.

The case manager observes that the husband and wife appear completely devoted to each other. They both tell her they don't want to be separated, which the case manager knows is a possibility if they go to a nursing home. They also tell the case manager they want to return to their daughter/caregiver's home.

After the assessment, the case manager concludes that she cannot justify a three-night hospital stay for the couple. However, she can't legally send the couple home because of the pending court order against the daughter/caregiver.

A temporary solution

Taking a risk, the case manager calls her director and asks for approval to let the couple stay in the ED overnight. This seems like the only choice because the couple cannot be sent home, they do not meet the hospital level of care, and a nursing home is not an option at this time.

The outcome

The case management director allows the couple to stay the night in the ED. Meanwhile, the case manager begins her investigation into all aspects of the case. A call to Elder Protective Services reveals that investigators can't find a case against the daughter/caregiver. However, even though the caregiver has been cleared, the pending court order still remains as a barrier to the couple returning home.

The next day, the daughter/caregiver goes to court and receive an order for protective custody. After a 24-hour ED stay, the case manager discharges the couple with their consent to their home.

Resources

Elder Services contact information:

_____

_____

Visiting nurses association contact information:

_____

_____

Hospital legal department contact information:

_____

_____

Elder Protective Services contact information:

_____

_____

Other resources:

_____

_____

HAL MODEL ASSESSMENT
For complex case management

H = High to very effective (score of >75%)
A = Average to moderately effective (score of 50%–75%)
L = Low to minimally effective (score of <50%)

Professional comfort (PC-1)
H = 25% A = 15% L = 5%

Professional objectivity
Personal values and ethics
Cultural and religious influence
Life's experiences and maturity
Personality type
Family history/dynamics

PC-1 score = _____

Professional competency (PC-2)
H = 25% A = 15% L = 5%

Clinical knowledge and skills
Professional training and education
Licensure and certification/code of ethics
Resource knowledge and management
Skills of your manager or supervisor
Case experiences/patients and populations

PC-2 score = _____

Consultation (C-1)
H = 25% A = 15% L = 5%

Mentor/mentorship
Supervision/case conferences
Whom you counsel/seek counsel from

C-1 score = _____

Collaboration (C-2)
H = 25% A = 15% L = 5%

Interdisciplinary/multidisciplinary meetings
Teamwork for continuity of care
Team up for desired goals

C-2 score = _____

Score: PC-1 + PC-2 + C1 + C2 = _____%

A case manager thinks outside the box when planning discharge for uninsured patient

The problem

Juan, a 43-year-old father of two, came to the United States from the Caribbean with his wife three years ago. Both Juan and his wife are illegal immigrants; however, they have obtained regular employment, established themselves in their community, and become active members in their church.

Juan is hospitalized because of a perforated bowel secondary to ulcerative colitis. His bowel is extensively damaged, and reanatomosis is not possible at this time. A colostomy is the only surgical option. Even if surgeons can repair the bowel later, it is unclear whether any function remains. Therefore Juan's nutritional intake will consist of daily infusions of total parenteral nutrition (TPN) costing $150 a day.

At the beginning of his hospital stay, Juan's physician was not sure he would even survive, but after two acute episodes requiring stays in the intensive care unit, it becomes clear he is on the road to recovery.

The case manager's approach

The case manager begins planning for Juan's discharge by examining all of the options available for this uninsured patient. The state's free care program covers Juan's hospital care, but this coverage does not extend after discharge. The case manager quickly learns there is no state program that will fund Juan's healthcare services beyond his hospital care.

The case manager assesses the family's commitment and potential financial resources. The family is completely devoted to Juan and assures the case manager that they will provide care at home. The case manager then secures a commitment from the local visiting nurses association (VNA) to donate two visits to the family to teach them how to care for Juan and to assist with the transition from hospital to home. The VNA also agrees to be on-call for any acute patient care issues. The one barrier that remains is the exorbitant cost of the TPN, which Juan's family cannot afford.

The outcome

The case manager and the family approaches Juan's church. The congregation holds a fundraiser and generates enough money to cover six months of infusion services. To maximize the church's donation, the case manager asks the hospital pharmacy if it can prepare the TPN at cost. Once the pharmacy agrees, the donation funds cover eight months of infusion therapy, just enough time before the patient will be readmitted for surgery to reanatomose his bowel.

Because of its license, the pharmacy can only distribute the medication within the hospital, so the family has to bring Juan in to the infusion clinic every day to have the TPN dispensed and the administration started. The case manager compares the cost of the outpatient infusion clinic to the cost of a continuous eight-month hospital stay, and persuades the hospital administration to cover the cost of the clinic visits.

The discharge plan, although complex, did end up meeting the needs of the patient. Eight months later the patient is readmitted for bowel surgery.

Resources

State free care contact information:

_____

_____

Visiting nurses association contact information:

_____

_____

Local religious groups and resources:

_____

_____

Other resources:

_____

_____

HAL MODEL ASSESSMENT
For complex case management

H = High to very effective (score of >75%)
A = Average to moderately effective (score of 50%–75%)
L = Low to minimally effective (score of <50%)

Professional comfort (PC-1)
H = 25% A = 15% L = 5%

Professional objectivity
Personal values and ethics
Cultural and religious influence
Life experiences and maturity
Personality type
Family history/dynamics

PC-1 score = _____

Professional competency (PC-2)
H = 25% A = 15% L = 5%

Clinical knowledge and skills
Professional training and education
Licensure and certification/code of ethics
Resource knowledge and management
Skills of your manager or supervisor
Case experiences/patients and populations

PC-2 score = _____

Consultation (C-1)
H = 25% A = 15% L = 5%

Mentor/mentorship
Supervision/case conferences
Whom you counsel/seek counsel from

C-1 score = _____

Collaboration (C-2)
H = 25% A = 15% L = 5%

Interdisciplinary/multidisciplinary meetings
Teamwork for continuity of care
Team up for desired goals

C-2 score = _____

Score: PC-1 + PC-2 + C1 + C2 = _____%

A noncompliant patient incurs extreme costs and extended LOS

The problem

In July, an illegal immigrant named Maria is admitted to the hospital. She uses an alias and a false Social Security number during her hospital stay because she is afraid she will be reported to the Office of Immigration and possibly be deported.

Unfortunately, during her hospital stay, Maria is diagnosed with an aggressive form of Hodgkin's disease, and upon discharge she is referred to the local Community Health Center. Maria visits the center where staff set a chemotherapy regimen and refer her to the Community Cancer Center.

During her stay in the hospital, she never revealed her real identity. Therefore, the case manager never saw the need for postdischarge follow-up to ensure she keeps her appointments and follows her treatment regimen. However, follow-up is essential for this patient because of her mistrust of the health system and her reluctance to speak with anyone who could report her immigrant status.

Maria never shows up for any of her chemotherapy appointments and, as a result requires a second admission to the hospital eight months later. She is admitted directly to the intensive care unit with a serious exacerbation of her Hodgkin's disease. When she is admitted she uses a second false name and Social Security number. However due to the severity of her illness, one of her friends reveals her real identity, and discloses that Maria never received chemotherapy.

The case manager's approach

Once properly informed, the case manager works with the financial counselor to complete a free care application using the patient's correct information.

The first day after discharge, the case manager calls Maria and learns that her phone has been disconnected. Luckily, before discharge, she had identified a friend who agreed to act as a sponsor for Maria. She quickly contacts Maria's sponsor to obtain her new phone number.

In the end, Maria's sponsor is essential to her compliance and ultimate success. Her friend makes sure she keeps all her chemotherapy appointments and, fortunately, Maria goes into remission.

The outcome

Ultimately, this catastrophic case results in a 58-day length of stay and costs more than $55,000.

As the case manager looked back at the high resource utilization of this case, she realizes that one manager dedicated solely to high-risk patients could have prevented this admission as well as other similar patient situations.

Maria was at high risk for noncompliance from the point of her first admission. If the facility develops a new case manger role that follows the high-risk patient from the hospital to the community, the patient's compliance to his or her treatment plan can be guaranteed.

Many patients could benefit from a high-risk case manager who could bridge intervention and care coordination from hospital to home to outpatient care. High-risk patients who could be followed by this program include the frail elderly, patients with complex or chronic illnesses, noncompliant patients, the mentally ill, immigrant, indigent, uninsured or minimally insured patients, those living alone or without a significant other, and those who suffer from head injuries but live independently.

Hospital administrators approve of the case manager's proposal for a high-risk case manager and allow her a three-month trial period. In-hospital and emergency department case managers refer patients to this new case manager. After three months, the facility's high-risk case management pilot demonstrates that this new position decreased readmission rates and increased patient satisfaction.

Resources

State free care contact information:

_____

_____

Other area high-risk case managers:

_____

_____

Other resources:

_____

_____

HAL MODEL ASSESSMENT
For complex case management

H = High to very effective (score of >75%)
A = Average to moderately effective (score of 50%–75%)
L = Low to minimally effective (score of <50%)

Professional comfort (PC-1)
H = 25% A = 15% L = 5%

Professional objectivity
Personal values and ethics
Cultural and religious influence
Life experiences and maturity
Personality type
Family history/dynamics

PC-1 score = _____

Professional competency (PC-2)
H = 25% A = 15% L = 5%

Clinical knowledge and skills
Professional training and education
Licensure and certification/code of ethics
Resource knowledge and management
Skills of your manager or supervisor
Case experiences/patients and populations

PC-2 score = _____

Consultation (C-1)
H = 25% A = 15% L = 5%

Mentor/mentorship
Supervision/case conferences
Whom you counsel/seek counsel from

C-1 score = _____

Collaboration (C-2)
H = 25% A = 15% L = 5%

Interdisciplinary/multidisciplinary meetings
Teamwork for continuity of care
Team up for desired goals

C-2 score = _____

Score: PC-1 + PC-2 + C1 + C2 = _____%

Helping a noncompliant patient with both schizophrenia and diabetes manage his health

The problem

Peter, a 50-year-old male, schizophrenic (not acute stage) Navy retiree, lost half of one foot from diabetes and poor diet. In 1999, he failed to take his oral medication as directed. His problem escalated such that he needs insulin, but he won't always do his fingersticks, and sometimes his supplies are low.

Peter is later admitted to the hospital for hypoglycemia and to control his sugars. Peter's case manager begins to build trust from the opening visit. She tells him she is always available for him if he needs assistance. He is excited to have someone help him with his treatment plan, but despite his good intentions, he has trouble with compliance because of his schizophrenia.

The case manager's approach

The case manager takes the following actions in this case:

☆ **Tap into community services:** The case manager sets Peter up with the local diabetic association support group.

☆ **Restock his supply:** The case manager provides Peter with more strips and glucometers and makes sure he understands when and why he needs to use them.

☆ **Calls:** The case manager calls Peter twice a week at first, then checks in with his primary care doctor and the diabetic educator at the hospital to evaluate his progress.

☆ **Transition:** With schizophrenic cases, this is a critical point. Peter isn't an acute patient in need of hospitalization, but he wrestles daily with his progress. Sometimes he feels better and wants to stop his medicines. Case managers must give the patient more independence while stepping up communication with the providers and doing more behind-the-scenes checking. The case manager on this case checks Peter's records more often, looking at his hemoglobin, kidneys, and other lab work.

The case manager tells Peter's primary care physician that he qualifies under the TriCare government insurance policy for home health visits. This is critical in helping Peter make more progress.

A social worker visits his home to make sure it is well lit and safe, and to make a list of necessary equipment, such as handrails or special toilets.

Because of Peter's neuropathy, a condition common in diabetics that leads to high blood glucose damage in nerve endings, causing a loss of balance, the case manager also facilitates a physical therapy (PT) visit. The PT will help Peter with his activities of daily living.

The outcome

Today, Peter remains in compliance with his medications and is doing well with the help of a new diabetes education program at the hospital called disease management drop-ins. The program is set up as follows:

- Patients report to a hospital conference room monthly
- Stations are set up to give patients a one-on-one review of their disease management from specialists for whom they would usually have to wait months to see (i.e., nutritionist, pharmacist, case manager)
- Patients are checked at a foot station for extremity damage

At the drop-in, the case manager and other specialists talk about transportation issues, access to care, and the patient's progress on the care plan.

Resources

Community support groups:

_____

_____

Local home health agencies:

_____

_____

Medical equipment supply resource:

_____

_____

Other resources:

_____

_____

HAL MODEL ASSESSMENT
For complex case management

H = High to very effective (score of >75%)
A = Average to moderately effective (score of 50%–75%)
L = Low to minimally effective (score of <50%)

Professional comfort (PC-1)
H = 25% A = 15% L = 5%

Professional objectivity
Personal values and ethics
Cultural and religious influence
Life experiences and maturity
Personality type
Family history/dynamics

PC-1 score = _____

Professional competency (PC-2)
H = 25% A = 15% L = 5%

Clinical knowledge and skills
Professional training and education
Licensure and certification/code of ethics
Resource knowledge and management
Skills of your manager or supervisor
Case experiences/patients and populations

PC-2 score = _____

Consultation (C-1)
H = 25% A = 15% L = 5%

Mentor/mentorship
Supervision/case conferences
Whom you counsel/seek counsel from

C-1 score = _____

Collaboration (C-2)
H = 25% A = 15% L = 5%

Interdisciplinary/multidisciplinary meetings
Teamwork for continuity of care
Team up for desired goals

C-2 score = _____

Score: PC-1 + PC-2 + C1 + C2 = _____%

A comatose stroke patient with no significant other, family, or friends

The problem

A 64-year-old female presents to the emergency department on a Sunday evening with med-sternal chest pain radiating down her right arm and up into her jaw. An electrocardiogram reveals changes consistent with an inferior wall myocardial infarction. Two sets of cardiac enzymes are ordered, and the patient is admitted to the cardiac telemetry unit. The patient has comorbidities including diabetes, hypertension, and slight renal involvement.

The admission clerk acquires the patient's name, address, and Social Security number. The patient claims she has no insurance, as well as no family or friends. She says she lives alone in her parents' home, both of whom are deceased. The home is still in their name, and the patient has not taken any steps to convert the deed over to her name.

On her first night in the hospital, the patient has a massive stroke, so the case manager is never able to assess her. The patient is now comatose, intubated, placed on a ventilator, and moved to the intensive care unit. A neurology consult is called, and the prognosis is unclear. The physician orders a magnetic resonance imaging, but the patient is too unstable to move.

The case manager's approach

The case manager views this case as high risk because of the complexity caused by the absence of significant others, the potential need to seek guardianship, and the lack of an identified source of insurance. Anticipating what is needed, the case manager

- teams up with the social worker on day one, and together they search for a significant other.
- files a free care application with the state.
- informs the hospital's legal department about the steps she is taking to avoid filing for guardianship. The case manager figures she has a week to locate someone who knows the patient before a guardian will be needed to determine whether the patient should have a tracheostomy.

The case manager notifies her director about this case, and because it is high risk, the team assigns increased case manager/social worker resources to the patient. Together, they agree that the patient needs appropriate representation. The team also identifies the ethics committee as a potential resource because the case manager may need to consider end-of-life measures. Overall, the utilization of clinical resources matches the prognosis.

The case manager/social worker team starts by requesting that the police speak to the patient's neighbors.

Tip: Once you pursue guardianship, your hospital's lawyers can request permission of the judge to go into the patient's house, but again, the legal process will not start for approximately one week. The police confirm that the patient is a recluse; no other information is obtained.

The outcome

The guardianship petition is initiated on day seven because the tracheostomy is planned for day 10 and no significant others are identified. A lawyer in the community is asked to accept guardianship in the absence of family or friends. This process normally takes several weeks, but it is expedited because of the proactive work of the case manager and the urgency of the treatment.
The hospital lawyer also appeals to the judge to permit the police to gain entry to the patient's house. On doing so, a card from a friend is found along with the patient's managed care insurance policy. When the case manager contacts the friend, an entire network of distant family and friends is found. They quickly come to the patient's side to provide support for the remainder of the stay.

Resources
State free care contact information:

_____

_____

Hospital legal department contact information:

_____

_____

Hospital Ethics Committee contact information:

_____

_____

Local police contact:

_____

_____

Other resources:

_____

_____

HAL MODEL ASSESSMENT
For complex case management

H = High to very effective (score of >75%)
A = Average to moderately effective (score of 50%–75%)
L = Low to minimally effective (score of <50%)

Professional comfort (PC-1)
H = 25% A = 15% L = 5%

Professional objectivity
Personal values and ethics
Cultural and religious influence
Life experiences and maturity
Personality type
Family history/dynamics

PC-1 score = _____

Professional competency (PC-2)
H = 25% A = 15% L = 5%

Clinical knowledge and skills
Professional training and education
Licensure and certification/code of ethics
Resource knowledge and management
Skills of your manager or supervisor
Case experiences/patients and populations

PC-2 score = _____

Consultation (C-1)
H = 25% A = 15% L = 5%

Mentor/mentorship
Supervision/case conferences
Whom you counsel/seek counsel from

C-1 score = _____

Collaboration (C-2)
H = 25% A = 15% L = 5%

Interdisciplinary/multidisciplinary meeting
Teamwork for continuity of care
Team up for desired goals

C-2 score = _____

Score: PC-1 + PC-2 + C1 + C2 = _____%

Russian woman discharged early with nursing staff help

The problem

Natasha, 55, travels from Russia to the United States in March to visit her daughter. During her visit, she falls and breaks her hip. Her daughter takes her to a major medical center where she is admitted.

Natasha has limited Medicaid, which means her hospital stay is covered, but she is not eligible for coverage for her care beyond the hospital visit. The hospital cannot discharge Natasha if she is not safe. "It's a catch-22," says the case manager. "If you keep the patient, the hospital is not paid. But if you discharge the patient early, then the hospital is liable."

Natasha's daughter is very devoted and willing to care for her mother in her home. She speaks English well, so language is not as large a barrier as it could have been. Natasha requires rehabilitation before the case manager can set any care plans, regardless of insurance.

The case manager's approach

The case manager arranges a discharge-planning meeting early on in Natasha's visit. All the disciplines caring for Natasha attend, and everyone agrees that she needed at least two weeks of rehab at a post-acute level.

The physical therapist (PT) offers to develop the post-acute rehab care plan; however, due to limited staffing in the PT department, she says they cannot fully operationalize the intensity of services. The case manager collaborates with the nurse manager to devise a plan.

The outcome

Nursing staff decide to help meet the physical-therapy care expectations. It works: In 10 days the patient shows a remarkable response. Natasha is discharged to her daughter's care two days earlier than scheduled.

Before discharge, the case manager contacts a local visiting nurse home care agency. The agency agrees to donate several visits to help Natasha in light of her limited insurance. It's often difficult to convince home care agencies to donate visits because once the home care agency goes in, it is responsible for the case if she needs further care. Luckily, for the case manager and Natasha, the agency agreed.

Resources

Hospital interpreter services contact information:

_____

_____

Visiting nurse home care agency contact information:

_____

_____

Local respite organization for caregivers:

_____

_____

Other resources:

_____

_____

HAL MODEL ASSESSMENT
For complex case management

H = High to very effective (score of >75%)
A = Average to moderately effective (score of 50%–75%)
L = Low to minimally effective (score of <50%)

Professional comfort (PC-1)
H = 25% A = 15% L = 5%

Professional objectivity
Personal values and ethics
Cultural and religious influence
Life experiences and maturity
Personality type
Family history/dynamics

PC-1 score = _____

Professional competency (PC-2)
H = 25% A = 15% L = 5%

Clinical knowledge and skills
Professional training and education
Licensure and certification/code of ethics
Resource knowledge and management
Skills of your manager or supervisor
Case experiences/patients and populations

PC-2 score = _____

Consultation (C-1)
H = 25% A = 15% L = 5%

Mentor/mentorship
Supervision/case conferences
Whom you counsel/seek counsel from

C-1 score = _____

Collaboration (C-2)
H = 25% A = 15% L = 5%

Interdisciplinary/multidisciplinary meeting
Teamwork for continuity of care
Team up for desired goals

C-2 score = _____

Score: PC-1 + PC-2 + C1 + C2 = _____%

Seizure disorder patient noncompliant with medications

The problem

Roger is a retired policeman with a history of seizure disorders. His seizures are difficult to manage, therefore repeated admissions are needed to determine and regulate the best therapeutic dosage for his anticonvulsants. Despite his physician's effort to regulate his medication, Roger has a history of frequent readmissions to a local hospital.

Usually the duration between each admission is at least three months, but recently the frequency has increased. During his most recent admission his case manager is concerned because Roger had shown up on her report for "readmissions in less than 31 days."

The number of patients who are readmitted in less than 31 days after discharge is a quality indicator measured and monitored by all the case manages in her department. The measurement of this indicator is required by the Joint Commission on Accreditation of Healthcare Organizations, and is a quality concern for any case manager. Repeated hospital readmissions occurring shortly after discharge can be the result of several serious issues. For example, it might indicate that the patient was discharged prematurely or that the discharge arrangements, set up by the case manager, were not adequate. It could also indicate that the patient's condition was complex or that the patient did not comply with the treatment regimen. In fact, readmission can be a red flag to the case manager and suggests that this patient falls into the high-risk category, requiring additional scrutiny when managing his or her case and discharge.

The case manager's approach

Roger's case manger is concerned about the number of readmissions and speaks to one of her colleagues about the case. Her colleague knows the patient and shares her impressions that Roger is noncompliant with his anticonvulsants. "He takes them for a while, and then he just stops," she says. Armed with that information, the case manager decides to conduct a high-risk screen of Roger.

"I noticed you were just discharged two weeks ago," she says to Roger. "Can you tell me about that discharge and what it was like for you while you were home?" At first Roger doesn't offer any critical information, until he starts speaking about his medications. Roger shows he understands his illness, and he sounds like an expert when describing the purpose and schedule for taking his medication. He tells her how important his medications are and that he always tries to take them on time. The case manager is baffled—it is clear that compliance is not the issue. "I am a proud man," he says, "so it is hard for me to tell you this, but I can't always afford my medications." Roger continues, "so, when I can't afford them, I just don't take them. It is as simple as that."

The outcome

Roger's case manager immediately starts to research a pharmacy benefit for him. His managed care insurance policy is limited and doesn't provide any coverage. Not ready to give up, the case manager continues to inquire about the patient's history and finds out the patient was a veteran. Roger supplies all the necessary information about his service in the Korean War. Finally, when Roger is discharged, his veteran benefits are in place, which include an adequate pharmacy benefit to cover the cost of his medications. The case manager also arranges for a community case manager to follow Roger for a period of time to support his transition to home.

Resources

Methods for screening a high-risk patient:

_____

_____

Pharmacy benefit resources:

_____

_____

Veteran's benefit information resources:

_____

_____

Area community case manager contact information:

_____

_____

Other resources:

_____

_____

HAL MODEL ASSESSMENT
For complex case management

H = High to very effective (score of >75%)
A = Average to moderately effective (score of 50%–75%)
L = Low to minimally effective (score of <50%)

Professional comfort (PC-1)
H = 25% A = 15% L = 5%

Professional objectivity
Personal values and ethics
Cultural and religious influence
Life experiences and maturity
Personality type
Family history/dynamics

PC-1 score = _____

Professional competency (PC-2)
H = 25% A = 15% L = 5%

Clinical knowledge and skills
Professional training and education
Licensure and certification/code of ethics
Resource knowledge and management
Skills of your manager or supervisor
Case experiences/patients and populations

PC-2 score = _____

Consultation (C-1)
H = 25% A = 15% L = 5%

Mentor/mentorship
Supervision/case conferences
Whom you counsel/seek counsel from

C-1 score = _____

Collaboration (C-2)
H = 25% A = 15% L = 5%

Interdisciplinary/multidisciplinary meetings
Teamwork for continuity of care
Team up for desired goals

C-2 score = _____

Score: PC-1 + PC-2 + C1 + C2 = _____%

Adult patient with an eating disorder

The problem

Jean was diagnosed with anorexia at the age of 16. Today, 12 years later, she is still afflicted with this condition. When Jean is admitted, she weighs only 78 lbs, significantly less than her ideal body weight. Her primary care physician (PCP), who had cared for her since she was a child, writes her care plan that states Jean has to gain 12 lbs before discharge. The case manager encourages the dietician to visit the patient immediately to determine the patient's dietary preferences. In conjunction with dietary intake, the PCP orders total parenteral nutrition (TPN) infusions.

The case manager, Nancy, makes sure the patient understands every step of her care plan because she knows Jean will avoid eating when she could. Nancy knows this could be a tough case, and she feels like she has to monitor it closely to ensure the expected outcomes and the planned weight gain, while meeting the length of stay expectations.

The case manager's approach

After three days, Jean has only gained 2 lbs. Nancy investigates and determines that Jean is vomiting after some of her meals. Nancy then speaks with the PCP, and they include a psychiatric consult in Jean's plan of care. Nancy believes the psychiatrist should provide daily sessions; however, the psychiatrist believes that the patient's long-standing eating disorder will not be helped by his visits.

Two weeks pass with Jean still gaining little weight. Frustrated, Nancy seeks out the psychiatric case manager who also knows the patient. The psychiatric case manager points out that Jean has failed many treatment programs, and with cutbacks in state programs' funding, there are few eating disorder treatment options. Among the programs that do exist, most are geared toward adolescents and do not accept adult patients.

Nancy continues to speak with her colleagues and consult with the psychiatric service. She eventually teams up with the unit social worker. Together, they uncover a program in the local metropolitan hospital that will take Jean, but only if she is medically stable prior to her referral—meaning she has to gain more weight.

Nancy calls a family meeting and invites the PCP and all other members of the healthcare team. Everyone who attends speaks about how this admission is different from Jean's prior hospital stays. "It's like she has given up," one nurse says.

The healthcare team implements a plan that combines medical and mental health intervention, including mood elevators and frequent visits by a psychiatrist. Jean's family makes a commitment to visit the hospital more to provide support whenever they can, and nursing staff will consistently encourage, monitor, and measure Jean's nutritional intake.

The outcome
The plan begins to work, and after only 10 days Jean had reached her goal weight. A physical therapist starts working with Jean and uses exercises to promote steady walking. Now that she is stable, Jean travels by ambulance to the eating disorder program at a nearby hospital.

Resources

Local eating disorder programs:

_____
_____

Local eating disorder support groups:

_____
_____

Ambulance services:

_____
_____

Other resources:

_____
_____

HAL MODEL ASSESSMENT
For complex case management

H = High to very effective (score of >75%)
A = Average to moderately effective (score of 50%–75%)
L = Low to minimally effective (score of <50%)

Professional comfort (PC-1)
H = 25% A = 15% L = 5%

Professional objectivity
Personal values and ethics
Cultural and religious influence
Life's experiences and maturity
Personality type
Family history/dynamics

PC-1 score = _____

Professional competency (PC-2)
H = 25% A = 15% L = 5%

Clinical knowledge and skills
Professional training and education
Licensure and certification/code of ethics
Resource knowledge and management
Skills of your manager or supervisor
Case experiences/patients and populations

PC-2 score = _____

Consultation (C-1)
H = 25% A = 15% L = 5%

Mentor/mentorship
Supervision/case conferences
Whom you counsel/seek counsel from

C-1 score = _____

Collaboration (C-2)
H = 25% A = 15% L = 5%

Interdisciplinary/multidisciplinary meetings
Teamwork for continuity of care
Team up for desired goals

C-2 score = _____

Score: PC-1 + PC-2 + C1 + C2 = _____%

COMPLEX CASE #10 —————————————————————

Prostate cancer patient with severe anxiety

The problem

R.J. is a 40-year-old patient with prostate cancer. Nothing seems to be going right for him—his last chemotherapy treatment was delayed because the hospital had no beds open at the time of his appointment. R.J. is always extremely anxious about his condition, despite the fact that he has been told that his chances for survival are high.

The case manager follows R.J. during two hospital admissions and has not seen any improvement in his anxiety level. She notes that his anxiety is interfering with his ability to carry out self-care practices, and it affects his attention span and his retention during patient teaching sessions. The case manager knows she needs a plan for intervention to help his anxiety if she is to meet her length of stay target for this patient.

The case manager's approach

The case manager's first step is to call a family meeting to discuss R.J.'s problem. R.J.'s wife agrees with the case manager's assessment and says that she has tried to alleviate his anxiety, without success. The patient's parents and siblings also agree with the case manager's conclusion that R.J.'s mental state interferes with his ability to care for himself.

Armed with this information, the case manager calls a meeting with R.J.'s healthcare team to discuss the case. All members of the team are in attendance, including the physician, nurse manager, staff nurse, social worker, physical therapist, nutritionist, pharmacist, psychiatrist and, of course, the case manager. They review the entire case and the treatment course is agreed upon, and the case manager brings up the topic of the patient's anxiety.

The psychiatrist offers the idea of providing daily sessions with R.J., and the social worker suggests arranging for a recovered patient with the same diagnosis to visit R.J. The team accepts these recommendations. The nursing staff say they can provide a consistent approach to communicating with R.J., in which they will speak slowly and directly to him to promote understanding and learning. The nurses will also allow him to verbalize any feelings he has about his disease or his treatment. The case manger agrees to offer the patient as much control as she can during the development of his discharge plan.

The outcome

Once informed, the patient and his family agree to the plan the healthcare team established. Almost immediately, R.J. responds to the new elements in his care plan. The case manager notices that his anxiety decreases when he participates more in his discharge plan.

R.J. and his family agree to discharge to his home with a home care assessment. The patient feels ready for physical therapy, so it is included in the home care evaluation. The cancer survivor who visits R.J. in the hospital will continue to visit him after discharge. R.J. openly discusses his fears and concerns during his sessions with the psychiatrist, which will continue on an outpatient basis after discharge.

With all the pieces in place, R.J.'s chemotherapy is completed on time and discharge occurs at the time originally planned.

Resources

Community cancer support groups:

_____

_____

Local home health agencies:

_____

_____

Other resources:

_____

_____

HAL MODEL ASSESSMENT
For complex case management

H = High to very effective (score of >75%)
A = Average to moderately effective (score of 50%–75%)
L = Low to minimally effective (score of <50%)

Professional comfort (PC-1)
H = 25% A = 15% L = 5%

Professional objectivity
Personal values and ethics
Cultural and religious influence
Life's experiences and maturity
Personality type
Family history/dynamics

PC-1 score = _____

Professional competency (PC-2)
H = 25% A = 15% L = 5%

Clinical knowledge and skills
Professional training and education
Licensure and certification/code of ethics
Resource knowledge and management
Skills of your manager or supervisor
Case experiences/patients and populations

PC-2 score = _____

Consultation (C-1)
H = 25% A = 15% L = 5%

Mentor/mentorship
Supervision/case conferences
Whom you counsel/seek counsel from

C-1 score = _____

Collaboration (C-2)
H = 25% A = 15% L = 5%

Interdisciplinary/multidisciplinary meetings
Teamwork for continuity of care
Team up for desired goals

C-2 score = _____

Score: PC-1 + PC-2 + C1 + C2 = _____%

COMPLEX CASE #11

Patient with subdural hematoma becomes complex after poor discharge planning

The problem

Catherine survived a mild stroke seven years ago with minimal residual effect. She has a limp on her right side, making her unsteady on her feet, but she remains active. She attends many social events and has a strong network of friends.

One morning after having breakfast with friends, she slips on a restaurant's highly polished marble floor. She falls backward and hits her head on the marble. Feeling more embarrassed than hurt at that moment, Catherine rushes out of the restaurant and drives home alone. Once home, she calls her physician who tells her to go straight to the emergency department. Physicians perform a CT scan which reveals a massive subdural hematoma.

The case manager's approach

Catherine's entire family is at her bedside in the intensive care unit when the case manager first meets the patient. Her family is extremely devoted to her, especially her husband. They live in a condominium not far from the hospital, and he visits every day and caters to her every need. Based on her initial assessment and Catherine's strong family support, the case manager anticipates she will go home at discharge with no services.

Catherine does well as the hematoma slowly resolves over a two-week period, and she is moved to a medical unit. Catherine stays on bedrest for most of her stay, and she notices that the muscles in her legs feel stiff, especially on the right side.

When the nursing staff start to sit Catherine on the side of the bed, she tells them she is dizzy and feels she will be unsteady on her feet. The case manager has not kept up with Catherine's progress because she still has her original discharge plan in place.

As the discharge date draws closer, Catherine's daughter voices her concern that her mother has not been offered the option of rehab therapy. Catherine has Medicare, and her daughter knows her mother has rights as a Medicare beneficiary. The daughter also knows that her mother will not be safe at home.

"Don't you think, because my mother had a previous stroke and she was admitted after a fall, that she would benefit from rehab?," the daughter asks the case manager. The case manager, sticking to her original plan, says that she agrees that Catherine needs rehab, but that it will be provided in the home, and that Catherine's husband can provide the necessary support. Catherine's daughter then points out that her parents live in a townhouse with 20 steep and narrow steps that her mother will have to climb to get to her second-floor bedroom. "Do you think she is prepared in her current condition to climb those?" the daughter asks.

The outcome

The case manager is shocked that she has been caught so unprepared. Her rush to a quick judgment about the case, without a complete understanding of the patient's home life and the lack of an update on the patient's condition has led her to develop an inadequate discharge plan. Shortly before the patient's discharge date, the case manager starts at square one and completes an admission assessment to ensure she has correct information about the patient and to start screening for a rehab facility.

Because she jumped to conclusions and skipped several steps in the discharge process, the case manager causes a delay in treatment for the patient, as well as a delay in discharge and an increase in length of stay. Frustrated, the case manager knows next time she will be consistent in her daily practice and complete each step of the discharge process, including screening/assessment, goal setting, planning, implementation, monitoring, documentation, and patient transition.

Resources

Local rehabilitation facilities' contact information:

_____

_____

Other resources:

_____

_____

HAL MODEL ASSESSMENT
For complex case management

H = High to very effective (score of >75%)
A = Average to moderately effective (score of 50%–75%)
L = Low to minimally effective (score of <50%)

Professional comfort (PC-1)
H = 25% A = 15% L = 5%

Professional objectivity
Personal values and ethics
Cultural and religious influence
Life experiences and maturity
Personality type
Family history/dynamics

PC-1 score = _____

Professional competency (PC-2)
H = 25% A = 15% L = 5%

Clinical knowledge and skills
Professional training and education
Licensure and certification/code of ethics
Resource knowledge and management
Skills of your manager or supervisor
Case experiences/patients and populations

PC-2 score = _____

Consultation (C-1)
H = 25% A = 15% L = 5%

Mentor/mentorship
Supervision/case conferences
Whom you counsel/seek counsel from

C-1 score = _____

Collaboration (C-2)
H = 25% A = 15% L = 5%

Interdisciplinary/multidisciplinary meetings
Teamwork for continuity of care
Team up for desired goals

C-2 score = _____

Score: PC-1 + PC-2 + C1 + C2 = _____%

A diabetic patient with behavioral and mental issues

The problem

Ray, a 62 year-old widower with diabetes, is admitted to the medical unit in the county hospital. When his wife died, he was left the house and medical coverage with a popular managed care company. Despite the fact that Ray is well-established and has a house to live in, he chooses to live on the street. He is admitted because he does not have his diabetes under control and a lesion on his foot is not healing.

The staff nurses, as well as the case manager, find it difficult to handle Ray's personality. He is demanding, and he causes a commotion on the unit when he does not get his way. Other patients complain when Ray's behavior becomes more difficult to control. Also, Ray insists that he be taken outside in his wheelchair every day for fresh air.

The case manager's approach

The case manger is concerned about the patient's behavior, along with his frequent outbursts. Even more so, she is concerned about Ray's daily trips outdoors. It is unclear whether this practice is consistent with hospital policy and procedure. So she talks to her director. Together they find the hospital policy on taking a patient outdoors. Even thought the policy allows it, both the case manager and her director do not support this activity. If the payer recognizes that the patient is going outdoors every day, it might not consider Ray at hospital level and may deny payment for his stay.

The case manager tries to reason with the patient, to no avail. During a second trip to her director, the case manger requests discharge of the patient because she believes his activities are endangering the staff and the hospital.

Her director advises to keep the patient at the center of her decision-making. The director also tells the case manager to make a plan with the healthcare team and then progress the case to the point of discharge. "If you do what is best for the patient, then everyone will benefit," she says.

The outcome

The case manager has the patient's foot lesion and its care reevaluated and updated. She then follows up on the endocrine and nutrition consult. Nurses teach Ray about wound management, insulin control, and diet, so he can better manage his diabetes. Physical and occupational therapy implement a plan of care. Soon after, the patient is ready for discharge. However, Ray refuses to go home when he is about to be discharged.

The case manager refers him to a 24-hour shelter, which provides medical care. Finally happy, the patient is discharged in a chair car paid for by the hospital.

Resources

Homeless shelters that provide medical care:

_____

_____

Local chair car companies:

_____

_____

Other resources:

_____

_____

HAL MODEL ASSESSMENT
For complex case management

H = High to very effective (score of >75%)
A = Average to moderately effective (score of 50%–75%)
L = Low to minimally effective (score of <50%)

Professional comfort (PC-1)
H = 25% A = 15% L = 5%

Professional objectivity
Personal values and ethics
Cultural and religious influence
Life's experiences and maturity
Personality type
Family history/dynamics

PC-1 score = _____

Professional competency (PC-2)
H = 25% A = 15% L = 5%

Clinical knowledge and skills
Professional training and education
Licensure and certification/code of ethics
Resource knowledge and management
Skills of your manager or supervisor
Case experiences/patients and populations

PC-2 score = _____

Consultation (C-1)
H = 25% A = 15% L = 5%

Mentor/mentorship
Supervision/case conferences
Whom you counsel/seek counsel from

C-1 score = _____

Collaboration (C-2)
H = 25% A = 15% L = 5%

Interdisciplinary/multidisciplinary meetings
Teamwork for continuity of care
Team up for desired goals

C-2 score = _____

Score: PC-1 + PC-2 + C1 + C2 = _____%

Continuing education credit quiz

Complete the following quiz and evaluation and submit it to HCPro to receive your case manager continuing education credits. Instructions for receiving credits can be found at the end of the evaluation.

Complex case #1: Ethics consult helps convince a difficult physician to implement a plan of care

1. Besides the ethics consult, what other consult may have been helpful to establish the patient's recovery?
    a. Psychiatry
    b. Cardiology
    c. Neurology
    d. Gastrointestinal
    e. None of the above

2. Family meetings are helpful because
    a. All family members are informed and updated at the same time
    b. Questions are answered, and everyone hears the same thing
    c. The patient's entire healthcare team is usually present
    d. Plans are agreed on by a consensus
    e. All of the above

3. The medical advisor supported the case manager by
    a. Acting as a consultant for the case manager
    b. Intervening with the patient's treating physician
    c. Meeting with the family
    d. Stepping in and providing patient care
    e. a and b only

4. The ethics committee's role was to
    a. Advocate for the patient and family
    b. Provide conflict resolution
    c. Plan care
    d. Discipline the physician
    e. a, b, and c

5. This entire conflict could have been minimized or avoided if the patient had
    a. Communicated her wishes to her family
    b. Completed a living will
    c. Filed a healthcare proxy
    d. Any of the above

Complex case #2: Considering the patient's best interest, payment, and bed capacity while managing a case

6. A case manager's responsibility when suspecting elder abuse is to
    a. Report it to the director of case management
    b. Report it to Elder Protective Services
    c. Call the patient's neighbors and investigate the case
    d. All of the above
    e. a and b only

7. In the case study, the case manager informed the director and Elder Protective Services about the case. Who else should be informed?
    a. The social worker
    b. The hospital lawyer
    c. The patient's primary care physician
    d. The ED case manager
    e. All of the above

8. The couple spent the night in the ED. How should Medicare be billed?
    a. ED visit only
    b. Observation
    c. Ambulatory procedure
    d. Hospital level only
    e. None of the above

9. What should the case manager's documentation include?
    a. Every detail about this case, including who was informed
    b. Plan and actions taken, including involvement with Elder Services
    c. Outcome of case
    d. All of the above

10. What would you consider for discharge services?
    a. Nutrition consult
    b. Visiting Nurse Association (VNA) to complete a safety evaluation in the home for fall prevention
    c. Physical therapy home evaluation
    d. Occupational therapy home evaluation

Complex case #3: Case manager thinks outside the box when planning discharge for uninsured patient

11. Are illegal immigrants eligible for Medicaid?
    a. Not eligible under any circumstances
    b. Always
    c. Only in extreme life-threatening circumstances, and it is difficult to access these benefits
    d. After five days in the United States

12. Free care usually covers which of the following:
    a. Hospitalization
    b. Physician care
    c. Pharmacy costs
    d. Home care visits

13. The family in this case needs to be taught the following:
    a. How to change dressings
    b. How to check for vital signs (e.g., temperature, weight)
    c. How to meet the patient's nutritional needs
    d. How to check for signs of imbalance
    e. All of the above

14. Innovative strategies used by the case manager to acquire financial support for this patient include
   a. Church donations
   b. VNA donated visits
   c. Hospital paid for total parenteral nutrition (TPN)
   d. Outpatient visits billed to free care
   e. All of the above

15. What was another fairly reasonable option for the case manager?
   a. Keep the patient in hospital
   b. Pay for the care herself
   c. Work out a payment plan for family
   d. Transfer the patient to another hospital
   e. None of the above

Complex case #4: A noncompliant patient incurs extreme costs and extended LOS

16. What else could be criteria for a high-risk patient who was not cited in the case study?
   a. Patients on five or more medications
   b. Postoperative patients
   c. All patients receiving chemotherapy
   d. Postpartum patients
   e. All of the above

17. The most effective strategy this case manager used to ensure Maria's compliance was
   a. Visiting her at home
   b. Driving her to chemotherapy
   c. Calling her family
   d. Asking her friend to be her sponsor
   e. None of the above

18. What are the benefits of establishing a community high-risk case manager position?
   a. Collaboration with community health centers
   b. Reduction in readmissions
   c. Enforce appropriate utilization of the emergency department
   d. Assignment to a primary care physician
   e. All of the above

19. What are the evaluation criteria used to measure community high-risk case management?
    a. Decreased readmission rate
    b. Compliance with primary care physician (PCP) appointments
    c. Compliance with treatment and medication regimen
    d. Prolonged hospital stays
    e. a, b, and c only

20. To overcome the patient's mistrust, the case manager can consult a(n)
    a. Cultural advisor
    b. Interpreter
    c. Clergy, from the patient's place of worship if possible
    d. Family
    e. All of the above

Complex case #5: Helping a noncompliant patient with both schizophrenia and diabetes manage his health

21. This case study exemplified one of the most powerful tools that a case manager has, which is
    a. Patient trust
    b. Clinical expertise in an unrelated field
    c. Bus tokens
    d. Clothes for patients in need

22. What interventions did the case manager put into place in the community that promoted the patient's compliance to his treatment regimen?
    a. Connection with the local diabetic association
    b. Adequate medical supplies
    c. Postdischarge calls
    d. Follow-up up with community caregivers
    e. All of the above

23. The case manager followed which of the following organ and lab results?
    a. Renal function
    b. Hemoglobin
    c. Glucose level
    d. All of the above
    e. None of the above

24. What advantage did the case manager gain for the patient by uncovering his insurance benefits?
    a. Longer hospital stays
    b. Home health visits
    c. Free medical equipment
    d. Free medications
    e. None of the above

25. How would you describe the "disease management drop-in" program?
    a. Patients come when ever they want
    b. Patients must report to the hospital monthly
    c. Patients attend one on one reviews at stations
    d. Patients attend foot station
    e. All but a

Complex case #6: A comatose stroke patient with no significant other, family, or friends

26. What were the other factors that made this a high-risk case, besides absence of a significant other, guardian, and insurance?
    a. Critical illness
    b. Intubated on ventilator
    c. Unclear prognosis
    d. Unstable
    e. All of the above

27. Which of the items below were examples of resources sought out in this case?
    a. Police
    b. Neighbors
    c. Ethics committee
    d. Hospital lawyer
    e. All of the above

28. The case manager took a proactive approach to this case, as exemplified by
    a. Including the director early in the case
    b. Teaming with a social worker
    c. Applying for free care
    d. Excluding the physician
    e. a, b, and c only

29. Once guardianship is obtained, then
    a. Permission can be obtained to enter patient's house
    b. Treatments can be performed without consulting the guardian
    c. IV therapy can be withheld
    d. The physician can implement any therapy without advice
    e. None of the above

30. Locating the friend in this case revealed which of the following?
    a. Presence of family and friends
    b. The patient's favorite foods
    c. Healthcare proxy
    d. A living will
    e. None of the above

Complex case #7: Russian woman discharged early with nursing staff help

31. Identify the strategies for early discharge utilized in this case:
    a. The family kept informed of the plan from beginning of case
    b. Holding a discharge planning meeting early in the case
    c. The nurse manager and staff were involved in plan
    d. None of the above
    e. a, b, and c

32. Which of the following suggests to the case manager that the discharge plan could have a successful outcome?
    a. The patient's daughter was devoted and willing to care for her mother
    b. The insurance source
    c. The patient's health
    d. Physical therapy availability
    e. None of the above

33. Limited Medicaid can be defined as
    a. Hospital-level care only
    b. Postdischarge care only
    c. Ambulatory care covered
    d. Medical procedure and outpatient covered
    e. None of the above

34. What is the "favor" the home care agency provided?
    a. A falls prevention consult
    b. A donation of several visits
    c. Feeding
    d. Teaching of medications
    e. None of the above

35. When physical therapy (PT) was short staffed the
    a. Nursing staff provided PT
    b. PT plan was eliminated
    c. Occupational therapy took over
    d. Daughter provided the care
    e. None of the above

Complex case #8: Seizure disorder patient noncompliant with medications

36. The Joint Commission on Accreditation of Healthcare Organizations (JCAHO) request hospitals monitor which of the following for quality?
    a. High-risk patients
    b. Readmissions in 31 days
    c. Weekend discharges
    d. Midnight discharges
    e. None of the above

37. How is a readmission within 31 days described by the case manager in this case study?
    a. As a high-risk indicator
    b. As a red flag
    c. As a sign that the patient may be noncompliant with his prescribed therapy
    d. As a sign of a complex medical condition
    e. All of the above

38. The case manager in this case study uses which of the following to identify the patient's issues?
    a. The patient's explanation
    b. Documentation
    c. Trends
    d. The PCP's explanation
    e. a and c only

39. The case manager investigates why the patient is noncompliant and determines the reason is
    a. Anger toward the disease process
    b. Financial
    c. Lack of knowledge about medications
    d. Dissatisfaction with the side effects
    e. Too busy to take medications

40. The case manager solves this problem by
    a. Uncovering a vital resource—the patient's veterans benefits
    b. Teaching the patient about the importance of his medication
    c. Providing support with VNA
    d. Referring the patient to a psychiatrist.
    e. Speaking with his family

Complex case #9: Adult patient with an eating disorder

41. LOS might have been reduced if the case manager had
    a. Fed the patient herself
    b. Involved the social worker at admission
    c. Eliminated the psychiatric consult
    d. Decreased the calories in the TPN

42. Difficult cases become more manageable when
    a. Family meetings are held early in the case and repeated as needed
    b. PCP collaboration is present
    c. Community resources are investigated early
    d. Healthcare team members are informed of the cases progress
    e. All of the above

43. Select the true statement below.
    a. Eating disorder programs for adults are readily available
    b. Most insurance programs have extensive psychiatric benefits with approved long LOS
    c. Adult eating disorder programs have been cut back in most states
    d. Adults with eating disorders do not require support on discharge
    e. Adults with eating disorders are just trying to get attention and usually snap out of it

44. What is the role of the dietician in the case?
    a. Identification of dietary preferences
    b. Attended family meetings
    c. Consulted with PCP on adequate nutritional intake
    d. Assessed daily nutritional intake
    e. All of the above

45. Who else could have been helpful in this case?
    a. The pharmacist
    b. The neighbor
    c. The recovered anorexic adult patient
    d. The clergy
    e. All but b

Complex case #10: Prostate cancer patient with severe anxiety

46. Delay in the patient's chemotherapy could produce which of the following?
    a. Anxiety
    b. Stress response
    c. Loss of trust in hospital
    d. Questioning efficiency and organization of PCP
    e. All of the above

47. Select the intervention(s) that could be used to reduce the patient's anxiety.
    a. Regular visits by a psychiatrist
    b. The psychiatric case manager develops a care plan for nursing staff on the unit
    c. Family involvement
    d. A recovered patient visits
    e. All of the above

48. Signs that the patient's anxiety decreased were evident when he
    a. Began to participate in self-care
    b. Refused to participate in discharge plan
    c. Did not participate in patient teaching sessions
    d. Refused to eat
    e. Had a short attention span

49. Chemotherapy can be offered as
    a. Outpatient only
    b. Inpatient only
    c. Either inpatient or outpatient
    d. An at-home service
    e. None of the above

50. What services should you set up for discharge in this case?
    a. Home care assessment
    b. Cancer survivor visits
    c. PT
    d. Chemotherapy at home
    e. a, b, and c only

Complex case #11: Patient with subdural hematoma becomes complex after poor discharge planning

51. How could the case manager better manage this case?
    a. Complete an admission patient assessment
    b. Interview the family
    c. Consider the effect of the stroke on this admission
    d. None of the above
    e. a, b, and c

52. What is the significance of the patient's fall in the restaurant?
    a. No significance
    b. Potential indication of shift in physical abilities (i.e., high risk for falls)
    c. Rushing from one event to another
    d. Supportive devices for ambulation may be required
    e. b and d only

53. The patient complained that her leg muscles felt stiff. How should the case manager have responded?
    a. Ignore the comment
    b. Obtain a PT consult
    c. Request that the nursing staff practice range of motion exercises with the patient
    d. Encourage the patient to exercise in bed (e.g., push against foot board)
    e. b, c, and d only

54. What are the steps in the discharge process?
    a. Screening/assessment
    b. Goal setting and planning
    c. Implementation and monitoring
    d. Documentation and patient transition
    e. All of the above

55. Now that the case manager changed her plan for the patient, what's the best discharge plan?
    a. Send home with no services
    b. Send home with services
    c. Send to rehabilitation center for an approximate 10-day stay
    d. Long-term care placement
    e. None of the above

Complex case #12: A diabetic patient with behavioral and mental issues

56. What would you recommend is the best way to identify and implement a plan to manage the patient's behavior?
    a. Collaborate with the nurse manager and nursing staff
    b. Consult with psychiatry (e.g., psychiatrist, psychiatric clinical specialist and/or case manager)
    c. Collaborate with the patient's PCP
    d. Peer to peer consultation with expert case manager
    e. All of the above

57. The patient's decision to be discharged to a shelter despite the fact that he had a house must be supported by which one of the following?
    a. Checking with other family members
    b. Psychiatric consult establishing the patient's competency
    c. Validation by another case manager
    d. Detailed case management documentation
    e. None of the above

58. What do you expect the case manager would include in her admission progress note?
    a. The patient's functional status
    b. The reason for admission

c. Any preliminary assessed discharge needs

d. Functional deficits

e. All of the above

59. What would you include in the documentation concerning the patient's request to be discharged to a shelter?

a. A comprehensive description of the request, including patient quotes

b. A statement of competency from psychiatrist

c. A staff nurse explanation

d. Significant other(s) comments

e. All but c

60. What postdischarge appointments would you consider?

a. PCP appointment

b. Diabetic clinic

c. Wound clinic

d. Social worker

e. All of the above

Evaluation ————————————————————

Please complete this evaluation and return it with your CE quiz.

1. **Please indicate below how well you feel this activity met the learning objectives listed. Please provide a response for each learning objective.**

   At the end of this activity I will be able to do the following:

   • Describe strategies to manage complicated patient cases to balance cost and efficiency and reduce patient length of stay.
      Strongly Agree
      Agree
      Disagree
      Strongly Disagree

   • Assess my strengths and weaknesses using the HAL model.
      Strongly Agree
      Agree
      Disagree
      Strongly Disagree

   • Identify community resources and programs that are available for patients with complicated issues.
      Strongly Agree
      Agree
      Disagree
      Strongly Disagree

2. **Please circle the appropriate responses below to rate the quality of this educational activity:**

   This activity was related to my case management needs
   Strongly Agree
   Agree
   Disagree
   Strongly Disagree

The exam for the activity was an accurate test of the knowledge gained

Strongly Agree

Agree

Disagree

Strongly Disagree

The program avoided commercial bias or influence

Strongly Agree

Agree

Disagree

Strongly Disagree

This program met my expectations

Strongly Agree

Agree

Disagree

Strongly Disagree

3. **Will this learning activity enhance your professional case management practice?**

Yes

No

4. **What is your title?**

5. **I found the process to obtain my continuing education credits for this activity easy to complete**

Strongly Agree

Agree

Disagree

Strongly Disagree

6. **If you did not find the process easy to complete, which of the following areas did you find the most difficult?**

Taking the exam

Completing the evaluation

Understanding the instructions

Other, please specify

7. If you have any comments on this activity, please note them below.

8. To complete the evaluation and submit for credit, please fill in your name and address below:

Name:

Company:

Address:

City:

State:

Zip:

Thank you for completing this evaluation of our case management continuing education activity!

To receive your continuing education credits, please send the completed quiz and evaluation to:

Robin Flynn
HCPro, Inc.
200 Hoods Lane
P.O. Box 1168
Marblehead, MA 01945